WHOLE FOODS COOKING: RECIPES FROM VITAMIN A TO ZINC

A whole foods eating guide aimed at adopting a fresh and healthier
"standard American diet"

BY

KATY MOON, M.S.
COPYRIGHT 2008
ISBN: 978-1-4357-2953-7

WHOLE FOODS COOKING
TABLE OF CONTENTS

INTRODUCTION

Eating healthfully has never been more important. Killer diseases such as diabetes, heart disease and cancer are running rampant in this country. Sadly, other countries that are adopting the same lifestyle and eating habits as the United States have also seen these diseases on the rise in recent years. It also appears that a lot of scientific research is focused on disease management, rather than prevention. Most nutritionists agree that disease prevention is significant, achieved primarily from eating healthfully and exercising regularly.

Cardiovascular disease is the number one cause of death in America today. The American Heart Association (American Heart Association [AHA], 2006, Heart Disease and Stroke Statistics—2006 Update) states that "in 2003, one out of every 2.7 Americans died as a result of cardiovascular disease." According to their statistics, "more than 60% of young people eat too much fat, and less than 20% eat the recommended five or more servings of fruits and vegetables each day" (AHA, 2006, Heart Disease and Stroke Statistics—2006 Update). Therefore, eating a diet of fresh, wholesome food contributes to a healthier heart.

Cancer is the second most common form of death in the United States—it accounts for about every one out of four deaths. According to the American Cancer Society (American Cancer Society [ACS], 2006, Cancer Facts & Figures 2006), "most cancers do not result from inherited genes, but rather are the result from damage to genes that occurs during one's lifetime" (p.1). Specifically, the organization declares (ACS, 2006, Cancer Facts & Figures 2006), that "mutations may result from factors such as smoking, hormones, chemicals, sunlight and the digestion of nutrients within cells" (p.1). Like with heart health, nutrition is a key factor in protecting people from various forms of cancer.

Diabetes is also a major concern. More and more young people are becoming afflicted with the disease, and many medical professionals attribute the rise to poor nutrition and exercise habits. It is estimated (National Diabetes Information Clearinghouse [NDIC], 2005, Total Prevalence of Diabetes in the United States, All Ages, 2005) that:

> In 2005, seven percent of Americans, or almost 21 million people had diabetes, and it is currently the third-leading cause of death in the United States. Adults with diabetes are two-four times more likely to develop cardiovascular disease and/or have a stroke.

Also, Timothy Gower (2006) states that "forty million Americans are afflicted with *pre*diabetes (also called syndrome X, metabolic syndrome, or insulin resistance syndrome), which is when blood glucose levels are higher than normal, but not as high to be considered diabetes" (p. 51). It is well-known that obesity may cause both diabetes and high blood glucose levels, and many people become obese by eating fast and processed foods.

Processed foods contain items such as refined flour, high fructose corn syrup, artificial colors and flavors, as well as trans fats and preservatives. Trans fat is a dangerous, human-made product that is produced when manufacturers use partially hydrogenated oils in place of natural oils to extend the shelf life and add flavor to many types of processed foods. Usually, these are listed as some type of hydrogenated oil on food labels, and many fast foods restaurants fry food in this type of oil, although many are going "trans fat free" as a result of recent public awareness. In fact, trans fat is considered so dangerous to human health that the city of New York has banned trans fat from being used in its restaurants. Scientific evidence shows that consumption of saturated fat, trans fat, and dietary cholesterol raises low-density lipoprotein (LDL), or "bad" cholesterol levels, which increases the risk of cardiovascular disease. Also, eating these foods takes the place of more nutritious choices, which may also lead to the killer diseases mentioned earlier, and many more. Important to note is that even though saturated fat from animal products is natural, it can also be dangerous by clogging arteries and raising LDL cholesterol if it is consumed in excessive amounts.

What nutritionists and scientists have proven is that there are vital nutrients and disease-fighting compounds in natural, freshly prepared whole foods like vegetables, fruits, 100% whole grains and lean protein. In the last fifty years or so, Americans adopted a standard diet of fast, frozen or otherwise-packaged food, and have gotten away from buying fresh food from the grocer and preparing it at home. Important nutrients are stripped when food is packaged. Grains are bleached and refined and salt, sugar and preservatives are added so that items can be stored on a shelf and prepared later. This leads to a diet full of calories, fat, salt and chemicals, which makes people sick; and devoid of the very things that lead to thriving health—vitamins, minerals, fiber, water, freshness and believe it or not: flavor and variety. It is no controversy in the medical community that heart disease, cancer and diabetes are far more common than before processed food and preservatives were introduced in America.

To add to that problem, there is also an obesity epidemic in America today, affecting not only adults but also children. If adults do not change their kids' eating and exercising habits, their children will possibly develop one of many deadly diseases, or at the very least, have a lower quality of life. In fact, many children are now developing type 2 diabetes, which used to be referred as "adult-onset diabetes," but the terminology has changed as a result of the young population being stricken with the disease due to lifestyle. One of the contributing factors to illnesses related to the "convenient" standard American diet is that adults are overwhelmed with work and family obligations and are stressed out, leaving little time to exercise and prepare fresh, healthy meals.

The goal of this cookbook is to illustrate the importance of eating fresh, natural, whole foods and to help families incorporate vitamins and minerals into their diet, through simple food recipes in support of a healthier lifestyle. To accomplish this goal, this cookbook provides recipes that are rich in specific nutrients (usually containing more than one type of vitamin and mineral). It is organized by chapters covering all of the essential vitamins and minerals needed every day to ward off sickness and disease. Specifically, this cookbook highlights American diet classics with a healthier twist. As we are all aware, America is now considered a cultural melting pot, so why not adopt cuisine from other countries to contribute to a healthy diet and redefine the standard American diet? In the following chapters, we've included food from Mexico, Italy, Germany, Greece, Africa, Asia and the Middle East. Feel free to experiment as you realize that modifying your favorite recipes into healthy items is easy. This makes American eating much more interesting and healthy!

At the beginning of each chapter, the Dietary Reference Intakes (DRIs) from the U.S. Department of Agriculture (USDA) will be listed for each nutrient. This is the amount determined by the USDA to meet the needs of about 98% of adults (National

Agricultural Library [NAL], 2001, Dietary Reference Intakes:

Recommended Intakes for Individuals, 2001). These numbers will

provide a baseline, so that readers, along with healthcare providers,

can determine how much of each nutrient is needed. The USDA is

replacing what used to be the minimum requirement—the

Recommended Dietary Allowance (RDA)—with DRIs, since the

DRI includes the upper limits of nutrients, as well as adequate

intake for nutrients that do not currently have an RDA. The goal

of the USDA in defining DRIs is the amount needed to prevent

chronic disease such as heart disease, osteoporosis and certain

cancers, and will reflect more closely what top nutritionists

recommend (NAL, 2001). Since this is a more sophisticated

system, and the USDA outlines the needs for people of all ages, the

recommendation for adult men and women from age 19-70 will be

used in this cookbook, in order to streamline the data. For a

complete list of DRIs, refer to the website:

http://nal.usda.gov/fnic. Even though the government has come a lot farther with nutritional research and advocating healthy eating, there still remain some nutrients that do not have a DRI value (as shown in later chapters), but that are beneficial to health, so they are included in this book.

Every chapter will have one or more recipes that focus on the chapter's specific nutrient. Therefore, if a reader has nutritional deficiencies or a disorder due to malnutrition, this cookbook outlines what foods contain those vitamins and minerals that may be lacking in the diet. Conversely, a reader can become aware of what vitamins and minerals to consume in moderation, because too much of a good thing can also lead to health problems. In the case of vitamins in minerals, an excess of any nutrient usually leads to the lack of another important one, so a balanced diet is the goal. One of the world's first physicians, Hippocrates, put it best by stating, "Let food be thy medicine and medicine be thy food." Therefore, nutritious food is medicinal—supporting body systems discussed in later chapters as well as contributing to longevity.

It may seem daunting to change bad habits like eating mostly fast, prepared or packaged food, but once people learn how to use delicious natural flavors, the processed foods are not missed. Plus, there are ways to prepare unhealthy foods in a healthier form or eat them in moderation (i.e., see the yam fries recipe in Chapter Five, or the turkey reuben recipe in Chapter Nine). The recipes in the following chapters are not designed to lose weight—it is hardly a diet of deprivation, but one that will nourish the body with whole foods. Hopefully, too, this cookbook will show that even though it may require more effort to eat more natural, whole foods, the payoff of better health is priceless.

According to Molly Siple (2005), "ten of the most healing foods are asparagus, tomatoes, wild salmon, spinach, red wine, onions, blueberries, oranges, whole grains, and nuts" (p. 62-67). It should not be hard to incorporate foods like these into the diet. A beginner "healthy eater," can start to eat foods like those listed above by adding tomatoes to salads and sandwiches; sautéing spinach (see recipe, Chapter One) to serve with grilled chicken or fish; adding blueberries to cereal or yogurt; bringing an orange to work or putting one in a child's backpack for a perfect, portable snack. Likewise, baby carrots are portable and tasty, and can be blended up into the delicious carrot miso dressing shown in the first chapter.

This cookbook can be a helpful tool to help families get on track with better nutrition. The point is the population would not be as sick and overweight if they consumed food that lack incomprehensible ingredient lists. As mentioned previously, think wholesome, colorful, and fresh, and the food will be healthier and delicious.

CHAPTER ONE: Vitamin A/Retinol/Beta-carotene

USDA/DRI: 700-900 mcg per day

Vitamin A promotes good eyesight, including night vision, and maintains healthy skin, teeth, hair, mucous membranes, and skeletal tissue. It also supports the immune system. According to Dr. Haas (1992):

> By supporting the integrity of the mucous membranes, it helps fight infection and pollutants. It is also considered an antioxidant, which fights damage from free radicals. These harmful substances can lead to cancers, ulcers, atherosclerosis, high blood pressure and stroke. (p. 94)

While there is some risk for toxicity when too much vitamin A is consumed, the demand for it increases when a person is under stress, smokes, lives in a polluted environment or is pregnant or nursing. Signs of toxicity include fatigue, nausea, vomiting, headache, dizziness, blurred vision, and loss of body hair. The only known side effect of consuming too much vitamin A is

12

carotenemia, a harmless condition where the skin turns an orange color.

Night blindness and other eye problems may be caused by a deficiency in vitamin A. Also low levels of this vitamin may cause problems with immunity and cancer, such as breast, cervical, lung, prostate, throat and stomach. In addition, it can lead to skin, teeth, ear, and hair problems. One indicator of vitamin A deficiency is small red bumps on the back of the arms.

Food sources of vitamin A include apricots, cantaloupes, carrots, collard greens, chili peppers, leaf and romaine lettuce, mangoes, nectarines, peaches, pumpkin, spinach and sweet potatoes.

Sautéed Spinach with Garlic and Lemon

The spinach in this recipe provides vitamin A.

1 bunch of fresh spinach

2 cloves of garlic, minced

Half of a lemon, juiced

1 Tbsp. olive oil

Salt and pepper to taste

In a large saucepan, heat olive oil over medium heat. Add garlic and spinach; stir until spinach is wilted, about five minutes. Remove from heat and add lemon, salt and pepper. Serves two as a side dish.

Carrot-Miso Dressing over Leafy Greens

The carrots and lettuce in this recipe provide vitamin A.

1 head of leafy lettuce, such as romaine, green leaf, red leaf or butter lettuce, chopped

2 medium carrots

1-inch of peeled, fresh ginger

1 garlic clove

3 Tbsp. fresh lime juice

1 Tbsp. soy sauce

1 tsp. miso paste

½ cup peanut oil

Salt to taste

Blend carrots, ginger, garlic, lime juice, soy sauce, and miso paste (usually found in the refrigerated section next to other soy products) in a food processor until smooth. Stream peanut oil into the processor until the dressing is thinned. Toss the dressing with chopped lettuce, and add additional vegetables, grilled Portobello mushrooms and/or chicken breast, if desired. Serves four.

CHAPTER TWO: Vitamin B

USDA/DRI: Biotin: 30 mcg/day; Choline: 425-550 mg/day; Cobalamin 2.4 mcg/day; Folate: 1,000 mcg/day; Inositol: no DRI; Laetrile: no DRI; Niacin: 14-16 mg/day; Orotic acid: no DRI; PABA: no DRI; Pangamic acid: no DRI; Pantothenic acid: 5 mg/day; Pyridoxine: 1.3-1.7 mg/day; Riboflavin (1.1-1.3 mg/day); Thiamin: 1.1-1.2 mg/day

A family of fourteen vitamins and accessory nutrients (above) make up vitamin B. Sometimes these nutrients are listed in the ingredients on the packages of enriched grain products. Those are the breads and rice that have been bleached and the stripped of all of their nutrients, and then these vitamins are added back during the processing phase. Just like with other supplements, the vitamins and minerals are not as readily available to the body when produced this way, compared to 100% whole grains and brown rice.

As a whole, the vitamin supports many important body functions such as energy production, metabolizing amino acids and fatty acids, and assisting in red blood cell formation. It is helpful to reduce stress and has been shown to ease premenstrual syndrome. It also maintains healthy skin, hair, eyes, and mucus linings. Large amounts of vitamin B can be found in nutritional yeast; although some people are sensitive to this food product. Vitamin B can also be made in the large intestine. Bacteria, yeasts, fungi and molds all are able to make vitamin B. Antibiotics are contraindicative to B since they not only kill the bad bacteria that cause infection, but also the good bacteria that produce different vitamins in the intestines. This family of vitamins is absorbed easily and when the body has too much, it is easily excreted in the urine so there is really no concern about taking too much vitamin B. The consumption of refined flour, sugar, coffee, tea, nicotine and alcohol all deplete the vitamin in the body, so it is important to incorporate the vitamin in the diet if any of these products are consumed on a regular basis.

The most touted of the specific B vitamins are B-12 and folate (or folic acid). B-12 (cobalamin) helps in forming new cells, maintaining nerve cells and breaking down fatty acids and amino acids. It is found only in animal and dairy products so vegans and most vegetarians need to make sure to get an adequate amount. It also aids in nerve metabolism and supports balance.

Folate assists in new cell formation and protects fetuses from neural-tube defects, which is why all prenatal vitamins contain folic acid. It also helps generate red blood cells, builds muscle, promotes wound healing, and produces helpful chemicals in the brain and nervous system. In addition, it can reduce levels of homocysteine in the blood, which is a risk factor for heart disease and stroke. Good sources of folate are asparagus, avocados, broccoli, chilies, seeds, spinach, beans and orange juice.

One fact to note is that the family of B vitamins will compete with each other in the body for absorption; therefore it works best when consumed as a complete vitamin.

Food sources of vitamin B include beans, whole grains, collard greens, escarole, kale, leaf lettuce, mushrooms, nuts, peas, spinach, and Swiss chard.

Split Pea Soup

Ham contains many of the B vitamins. Split peas contain thiamin and folate, as well as smaller amounts of other B vitamins.

1 small ham hock

1 lb. split peas, rinsed

2 large carrots, chopped into small chunks

3 celery stalks, sliced into small pieces

½ onion, chopped into small chunks

2 garlic cloves, minced

2-32 oz. cartons of chicken broth

1 bay leaf

1 tsp. dried thyme

Salt and pepper to taste

Place all of the ingredients (except salt and pepper) in a large stock pot and bring to a boil. Reduce heat to low and cook for 2.5 hours or until vegetables are tender. Remove ham hock, let cool, remove meat and return shredded meat to the pot. Remove bay leaf and add salt and pepper, if needed. Serve with a healthy, high-fiber baguette or roll. Serves six.

Mexican Chicken Salad

Chicken is a source of niacin and B-6. Black beans contain folate, and the lettuce contains thiamin, riboflavin, folate and B-6. This recipe includes some healthy convenience foods, like the pre-made chicken and canned beans and corn.

1 rotisserie chicken, meat removed

2 heads of romaine lettuce, chopped

2 tomatoes, chopped into small chunks

1 avocado, cubed into small pieces

½ can pinto or black beans, rinsed and drained

½ can corn, drained

¼ red onion, sliced into half-moon shapes

½ cup low-fat cheese

Dressing:

1/2 cup all-natural real mayonnaise

2 Tbsp. lime juice

2 sun-dried tomatoes in oil or 1 Tbsp. tomato paste

1 tsp. each, dried cumin and oregano

Salt and pepper to taste

Blend the dressing ingredients in a food processor or blender until smooth. Toss all of the salad ingredients together with the dressing and serve. Serves six.

Beef and (Susan's Beans) Burritos

Beef and beans both contain vitamin B.

1 lb. dried pinto beans, rinsed

2 lb. beef brisket

1 onion, chopped into small chunks

2 garlic cloves, minced

1 cup low-fat Mexican cheese

8-all natural, high fiber flour tortillas

1 tsp. each, dried cumin and chili powder

Salt and pepper to taste

Salsa, recipe to follow

Rinse the beans, cover with cold water and soak overnight. When you are ready to cook, discard soaking water and place the beans and three cups of fresh water in a large stockpot. Boil for twenty minutes, then reduce heat to medium-high for a slower boil until tender, approximately two-three hours. During the last fifteen minutes of cooking, make a roux by browning a tablespoon of flour in a tablespoon of butter and add to the beans to thicken. Add salt and pepper to taste. Meanwhile, in a crock-pot or roaster, slow-cook the brisket, onions, cumin. chili powder and garlic for three hours or until the meat is very tender. Once the meat is cooled, shred it and place in a tortilla with beans, salsa and cheese, if desired. Serves eight.

Fresh Tomato Salsa

5 tomatoes, chopped into small pieces

1 jalapeno pepper, minced

¼ cup cilantro, minced

½ onion, chopped into small pieces

1 garlic clove, minced

One lemon or two limes, juiced

Salt and pepper to taste

Mix all ingredients and serve. Serves eight as a condiment.

CHAPTER THREE: Vitamin C

USDA/DRI: 75-90 mg/day

Many nutritionists believe that it would be safe and

beneficial to consume more vitamin C than the USDA

recommends. Vitamin C is an essential nutrient, which means that

it must be obtained from food and supplements because the body

does not make it on its own. Cooking can destroy much of the

vitamin C's properties (as is true of other nutrients), so this is

another important reason to incorporate fresh fruits and vegetables

into the diet. Vitamin C is an antioxidant vitamin and acts as a

detoxifier. It is used around the world as a cold prevention and

remedy, although its effectiveness in this manner is still

controversial and not conclusively proven. Many studies,

however, show vitamin C to support the immune system and along

with its antioxidant function, help to prevent infections and

diseases. It has also been shown to increase the production of

lymphocytes, which are the white blood cells that produce

antibodies and fight infection. According to Lieberman and
Bruning (1997):

> Even traditionalists such as the National Cancer Institute
> and American Cancer Society feel that the evidence is
> strong enough to warrant a diet high in vitamin C as a
> possible preventive measure [for cancer]. (p. 123)

Vitamin C has many additional benefits such as keeping
teeth and gums healthy, aiding in iron absorption, promoting
healthy connective tissue, producing collagen, and healing wounds.
Collagen is needed to give support and shape to the body and to
maintain healthy blood vessels. Vitamin C is also helpful in
thyroid hormone production and in cholesterol metabolism.
Deficiency in vitamin C can lead to the rare disease scurvy, which
causes gum inflammation and bleeding, poor wound healing,
resistance to infection, and possibly death. The disease is rare
today, but deficiency problems may still occur for those people
who never eat fresh fruits and vegetables. In addition to gum and

wound problems, a lack of the vitamin has been shown to cause digestive problems, bone fragility, colds, depression, allergies, ulcers, gallstones and may even lead to stroke and heart attacks.

Sources of vitamin C include avocado, broccoli, cabbage, cantaloupes, cauliflower, grapefruit, green and red peppers, Brussels sprouts, kiwi, lemons, limes, oranges, papayas, strawberries, tomatoes, dark leafy greens and sauerkraut.

Turkey Sausage with Potatoes and Sauerkraut

The sauerkraut, potatoes and onions in this recipe provide vitamin C.

5 turkey or other lean sausage links, preferably bratwurst, polish or spicy flavor

4 red potatoes, chopped into chunks

3/4 onion, chopped into ¼ half-moon shapes

1 Tbsp. olive oil

1 10 oz. jar of sauerkraut

Half of a bottle of beer

Brown the sausages according to package directions and set aside. Sauté the onions and potatoes in a large skillet for six-seven minutes. Add the remaining ingredients and the sausage to the skillet and simmer until the vegetables are tender, approximately thirty minutes. Serve with mustard, sour cream, or with a simple green salad. Serves four.

Greek Chicken with Zucchini, Sun-Dried Tomatoes and Feta Cheese

Lemons, onions and sun-dried tomatoes are sources of vitamin C.

2 lbs. chicken breast, cubed into 2" pieces

2 Tbsp., and 2 tsp. olive oil

One lemon, juiced

2 cloves garlic, minced

1 tsp. Greek seasoning

½ onion, chopped into small pieces

2 zucchini, chopped into small chunks

5 sun-dried tomatoes, sliced

½ cup feta cheese

¼ cup pitted kalamata olives, chopped

Salt and pepper to taste

Marinate chicken in the refrigerator with two tablespoons of olive oil, lemon juice, garlic and seasoning for at least two, and up to twenty-four hours. Remove chicken from the refrigerator and let rest at room temperature for another twenty minutes. Sauté chicken over medium heat until thoroughly cooked (about five minutes on each side) and set aside. In the same pan, cook the vegetables in two teaspoons of olive oil until softened, approximately eight minutes. Add chicken until reheated, mix with cheese, sun-dried tomatoes, and olives, if desired, and serve alone or with couscous recipe below. Serves four.

Couscous with Garbanzos and Pistachios

1 cup whole grain couscous

1 Tbsp. butter

½ cup canned garbanzo beans (chick peas), rinsed

¼ cup slivered pistachios

Pinch of salt

Bring one cup of water with butter and salt to a boil, add couscous and beans and remove from heat. Cover for five minutes until couscous is cooked. Fluff with a fork and add a handful of slivered pistachios. Serves four.

CHAPTER FOUR: Vitamin D

USDA/DRI: 15 mcg/day

Vitamin D is produced in the skin when it is exposed to sunlight. Cloudy or smoggy skies, darker skin tone and sunscreens all minimize the amount of vitamin D manufactured in the skin. The role of vitamin D is to help regulate calcium metabolism and utilize phosphorous, which along with other minerals, makes up the bone structure. Therefore, vitamin D promotes healthy bones. It also helps to maintain a healthy nervous system and heart, and has been shown to contain anticancer properties.

Too much of the vitamin may lead to toxicity problems such as calcification of soft tissues and arteries. Less problematic indicators like thirst, diarrhea, nausea, headaches and weakness are similar to sun poisoning, and Haas (1992) believes that sufferers of sun poisoning are actually experiencing vitamin D toxicity from overexposure to the sun and therefore, the vitamin.

Deficiency is more of a concern since many people do not get enough exposure from the sun because they live in a cloudy climate and/or use sunscreen. Also, older people and people with gastrointestinal diseases may not be able to absorb the vitamin which can lead to rickets (fragile bones) and/or osteoporosis (diminishing bones). A lack of the vitamin may also affect vision and hearing.

Sources of vitamin D include sunshine, liver, egg yolk, butter, mushrooms, and oily fish. Vitamin D is also added to some items such as milk and breakfast cereal.

Cobb Salad

Eggs provide vitamin D.

1 head of romaine or green leaf lettuce, chopped

1 large tomato, chopped into small pieces

1/8 red onion, sliced into half-moon shapes

1 avocado, cubed into small pieces

½ cup feta, blue or goat cheese, crumbled

2 hard boiled eggs, chopped into small pieces

½ carrot, peeled into curls

¼ cup canned julienne beets, drained

¼ cup canned garbanzo beans, rinsed

½ cup balsamic vinaigrette (recipe follows) or any other dressing

Toss together all of the ingredients and serve. Serves six.

Katy's Best Balsamic Vinaigrette

I've been told this is the best dressing for balsamic vinaigrette lovers, hence the modest name.

¼ cup extra virgin olive oil

¼ cup balsamic vinegar

1 garlic clove, minced

½ tsp. each: salt, pepper and dry mustard

Put all ingredients except oil into a wide-mouth jar. Slowly stream in the oil while whisking briskly to emulsify.

CHAPTER FIVE: Vitamin E

USDA/DRI: 15 mg/day

This vitamin is an important antioxidant whose purpose is to fight free radicals. As mentioned in Chapter One, these harmful compounds cause many degenerative diseases associated with aging and poor health such as heart disease and cancer. Because of this powerful benefit, vitamin E helps protect the body from carcinogens and toxins.

Frying, processing and cooking foods, as well as bleaching flour removes a lot of the vitamin E content of whole foods. As Haas (1992) states:

> The protective covering or germ part of the grains is what
> contains the E, and this is easily lost in the milling of flour
> or in the refinement of grains. For the vitamin E to be
> preserved, extraction of the oils from nuts and seeds must
> be done naturally, as by cold pressing, rather than by heat

or chemical extraction, used commonly in food processing.
(p. 101)

This is another reason this cookbook highlights eating 100% whole grains and whole foods rather than making meals from foods that are a processed version. Also, in this cookbook extra-virgin olive oil is used a lot, which is a healthy, monounsaturated fat loaded with vitamin E, so using this type of oil will help to incorporate the vitamin into the diet.

Vitamin E has been used to relieve menstrual and menopausal problems. Some studies have led researches to believe that a diet without enough vitamin E can lead to infertility. This is interesting since infertility seems to be on the rise, while the standard American diet is lacking in this vitamin. Vitamin E has also been shown to speed scar healing and promote healthy skin, as well as support the immune and nervous systems.

Food sources of vitamin E include unprocessed or cold pressed vegetable oil, such as extra-virgin varieties, asparagus, avocados, blackberries, chilies, corn, kale, kiwi, mangoes, nuts, spinach, Swiss chard, and sweet potatoes.

Roasted Asparagus with Parmesan

Asparagus and olive oil are sources of vitamin E.

1 bunch of asparagus, ends trimmed

¼ cup olive oil

½ cup shredded parmesan

Salt and pepper to taste

Preheat oven to 400°F. Toss asparagus on a cookie sheet with olive oil, salt and pepper. Sprinkle with parmesan and roast for ten-twelve minutes until tender-crisp. Serves four as a side dish.

Guacamole

Avocadoes are a source of vitamin E.

2 ripe avocados

½ cup salsa (recipe in Chapter Two, or buy prepared)

Juice of half a lemon

Salt and pepper to taste

Cut the avocados in half and scoop out avocado into a medium bowl. Add salsa, lemon juice, and salt and pepper. Mix together and serve with Beef and Bean Burritos (recipe, Chapter Two), or with baked tortilla chips as an appetizer. Serves six.

Corn and Zucchini Sauté

Corn contains vitamin E.

1 cup frozen or canned corn

2 zucchini or other squash, sliced into half-moon shapes

½ cup onion, chopped into small pieces

1 garlic clove, minced

2 tomatoes, chopped into small pieces

1 Tbsp. olive oil

Salt and pepper to taste

In a large skillet, sauté onion and garlic in the olive oil over medium heat for about two-three minutes. Add zucchini and sauté until tender, about six minutes more. Add corn, tomatoes and seasonings and heat through. Serves four people as a side dish.

Sweet Potato Fries

Sweet Potatoes contain vitamin E.

2 medium sweet potatoes, peeled

1½ Tbsp. olive oil

Salt to taste

Preheat oven to 450°. Cut potatoes into ½ inch wedges and toss with olive oil and salt in a medium bowl. Spread onto baking pan in a single layer and bake for 30-40 minutes. Flip once during cooking. Serves four.

CHAPTER SIX: Vitamin K

USDA/DRI: 90-120 mcg/day

Vitamin K is important in blood clotting. It is found in the food sources listed below as well as in the intestinal bacteria. Haas (1992) declares that "Vitamin K is absorbed from the upper small intestine with the help of bile or bile salts and pancreatic juices and then carried to the liver for the synthesis of prothrombin, a key blood-clotting factor" (p. 108). Newborn babies are injected with the vitamin at birth since their gastrointestinal tract does not start thriving until a few days after birth. This helps protect babies against wounds and promotes the blood-clotting ability. To that end, it can also be given to people of any age if there are problems with blood clotting. On the other hand, the blood thinning medication Coumadin was designed to specifically stop the action of vitamin K, to help reduce the incidence of blood clots in certain people. Deficiency may occur with antibiotic use, since antibiotics are designed to kill all of the bacteria in the body, even the beneficial form that produces vitamin K and provides other healthy benefits.

Food sources of vitamin K include items with bacteria such as yogurt, kefir and acidophilus milk. Alfalfa, Brussels sprouts, cabbage, escarole, kale, kelp, Swiss chard, spinach, turnip greens are also sources of the vitamin.

Spiced Lentils

This recipe contains yogurt, which is a source of vitamin K, and can be used as a topping in many dishes in place of sour cream.

1 Tbsp. olive oil

1 onion, chopped into small pieces

1 Tbsp. peeled ginger, minced

¾ tsp. each, salt and pepper

2 garlic cloves, minced

2 tsp. each: cumin and curry powder

1 tsp. ground coriander

2½ cups water

2 cups chicken broth

2 cups dried lentils

3 bay leaves

1 cup plain low-fat yogurt

¾ cup tomato sauce

Heat the oil in a stock pot over medium heat. Add the onion, ginger, salt and pepper and sauté for ten minutes. Add the garlic, cumin, curry powder and coriander, and stir together for one minute. Stir in the water, broth, lentils and bay leaves and bring to a boil. Reduce heat, cover and simmer for 1.5 hours or until lentils are tender. Discard bay leaves. Stir in yogurt and tomato sauce and simmer over low heat until heated through. Serve as a side dish or with warm, 100% whole wheat pita bread. Serves six.

CHAPTER SEVEN: Vitamin P

Vitamin P (no DRI) is also called bioflavonoids, and is the water-soluble component of vitamin C. It is helpful in the absorption of C, and its main function is to increase the strength of the capillaries. These tiny veins deliver oxygen and nutrients to the organs, tissues and cells and pick up waste and carry it through the veins and back to the heart. Capillary health is also important to protect us from infection.

Food sources of vitamin P include the white rind of fruits, citrus fruits, cherries, apricots, grapes, plums, blackberries, papayas, green pepper, broccoli, tomato and buckwheat.

Whole Wheat Veggie Pizza

This recipe contains wheat and tomatoes, which are sources of vitamin P.

Prepared wheat pizza dough or already-baked crust

½ cup Italian Tomato Sauce (recipe, Chapter Twenty-One) or

Pesto Sauce (recipe, Chapter Eleven)

8 oz. cremini mushrooms, sliced

½ of a green bell pepper, sliced into strips

½ cup onion, chopped into small pieces

2 garlic cloves, minced

1 bunch fresh spinach, washed and trimmed

1 cup low-fat mozzarella cheese

15 chopped sun-dried tomatoes packed in olive oil

Salt and pepper to taste

Preheat oven to 400°F. Meanwhile, sauté mushrooms, pepper, onions, and garlic in a medium skillet over medium heat until tender, about eight minutes. Add the spinach and seasonings and sauté until wilted, about five minutes. Roll out the dough into a pizza shape; place it on a pizza stone or other large baking sheet and top with sauce, cheese and vegetable mixture. Bake for fifteen-twenty minutes, until the crust is cooked (if using raw) and cheese is melted. Remove from heat and top with sun-dried tomatoes. Serves four.

CHAPTER EIGHT: Calcium

USDA/DRI: 1,000-1,200 mg/day

Approximately two percent of the body's weight is made up of calcium in the bones, teeth and other tissues. The nutrient is critical during infancy and childhood years as the skeletal system is forming, but it remains important to maintain a healthy structure once it is established. Bones not only serve as the physical support structure, but also as a reservoir for calcium. Other nutrients such as magnesium, phosphorous and vitamin D are required to absorb calcium and for it to function properly. Vitamin D, for instance, helps maintain the level of calcium in the blood, and is why most milk is enriched with this vitamin. According to Haas (1992), "one theory about multiple sclerosis correlates it with calcium and vitamin D deficiency in puberty" (p. 168). Calcium builds and maintains strong bones and teeth, regulates the heartbeat and other muscle contractions, helps with blood clotting, and is important in nerve transmission.

When there is not enough calcium in the diet, the body's intricate balancing system will draw it out of the bones to use for blood and cellular functions, which may lead to osteoporosis (diminishing bones). Low levels of calcium can also lead to osteomalacia (softening of the bones) and rickets (fragile bones). Unfortunately there is no reliable screening method to determine calcium levels in the body until a person begins to experience deficiency problems. Also, too much phosphorous from meat, soda and processed food, as well as certain medications like antibiotics, contraceptives and anticonvulsants can interfere with calcium absorption.

Regular weight bearing exercise like jogging and weight training has been shown to improve calcium absorption and utilization.

Food sources of calcium include dairy products, almonds, broccoli, escarole, fortified soy milk and juice, kale, seed, nuts, peas, beans, spinach, tofu and turnip greens. However, food items containing oxalic acid, such as spinach, chard and beet greens may interfere with calcium absorption so these items are not considered to be reliable sources of the mineral.

Noodles with Tofu-Peanut Dressing

Peanuts and tofu contain calcium.

16 oz. 100% whole wheat pasta

2 tsp. peanut or sesame oil

1 cup carrots, grated

2 scallions, white and most of green parts sliced thin

¼ cup cilantro, chopped

3 Tbsp. peanuts, chopped

Salt and pepper to taste

Lime wedges

Dressing:

½ cup all-natural peanut butter

½ cup low-fat firm silken tofu

¼ cup soy sauce

3 Tbsp. lime juice

2 Tbsp. brown sugar

3 garlic cloves, minced

¾ tsp. crushed red pepper flakes

Cook the pasta according to package directions. Meanwhile, combine all of the dressing ingredients in a blender or food processor and process until smooth.

After draining the pasta, rinse with cold water and toss with the oil. Add vegetables and dressing, and toss to coat. Serve with lime wedges. Serves four.

CHAPTER NINE: Chlorine/Chloride

USDA/DRI: 2-2.3 grams/day

Chloride helps regulate the body fluids such as stomach acid, and it helps maintain the body's acid-base balance. The kidneys will retain or excrete chloride in order to increase or decrease acid levels as needed. Too much of the mineral may cause problems with this balance, as well as fluid retention. Chloride may also help the liver to eliminate waste products.

As with the other minerals, chloride may be lost as a result of excessive vomiting, diarrhea or sweating, which will affect the acid-base balance in the body.

Food sources of chloride include salt, seaweeds, olives, rye, lettuce, tomatoes and celery.

Greek Salad

Lettuce, tomatoes, olives and salt contain chloride.

1 head romaine lettuce, chopped

2 grilled chicken breasts, sliced

2 tomatoes, chopped into small chunks

¼ red onion, sliced into half-moon shapes

½ cup feta or goat cheese

¼ cup pitted kalamata olives

½ peeled cucumber, chopped into small chunks

½ cup Greek dressing

Dressing:

¼ cup extra virgin olive oil

¼ cup red wine vinegar

Juice of ½ of a lemon

1 garlic clove, minced

½ tsp. each: salt, pepper and oregano

In a medium skillet or barbeque, grill the chicken over medium heat until cooked through (about five minutes on each side). Let the meat rest for five minutes, and then slice into strips. Place all of the dressing ingredients into a jar. Add oil last by slowly streaming it into the jar while whisking briskly to emulsify.

Toss all salad ingredients with dressing and serve. Serves four.

Turkey Reuben Sandwich

The salty sauerkraut and rye bread in this recipe contain chloride.

4 slices fresh, low-fat turkey breast deli slices

4 slices of 100% whole grain rye bread

2 slices Swiss cheese

¼ cup sauerkraut

¼ onion, sliced into half-moon shapes

1 tsp. olive oil

4 tsp. thousand island dressing

Grill onions in olive oil over medium heat until soft, about six minutes. Meanwhile assemble the rest of the ingredients on the bread, and add the onions when they are done. Makes two sandwiches.

CHAPTER TEN: Magnesium

USDA/DRI: 320-420 mg/day

Magnesium is important for nerve and muscle function as well as assisting in the body's absorption of calcium. Magnesium is involved in many enzymatic reactions such as those that produce energy and promote cardiovascular function. While calcium stimulates muscle contraction, magnesium relaxes muscles. Without magnesium, the vascular muscles would be tighter, which may lead to high blood pressure. The mineral is also thought to relieve premenstrual problems—perhaps through uterine muscle relaxation.

A deficiency in magnesium has been linked to high blood pressure, heart disease and kidney stones. In addition, according to Gower (2006), in a 2004 study at Harvard University, researchers "found that people with the highest intake of magnesium lowered their risk for diabetes by about one-third" (p. 52). This is important to note since the introduction to this book highlights diabetes as the third most common cause of death in America today.

Diuretic drugs, alcohol, caffeine and sugar all contribute to a loss of magnesium in the body. Because alcohol affects magnesium absorption, it is thought that hangovers may be a result of this interaction.

As with calcium, oxalic acid found in such foods spinach and Swiss chard can interfere with magnesium absorption, as can phytic acid in some grains. Also, as is the case with most nutrients, the processing and refining of grains and the oil extraction from nuts reduces magnesium content.

Food sources of magnesium include dairy products, meat, seafood, dried beans, green vegetables, nuts and seeds, soy, 100% whole grains, avocados and dried apricots.

Black Bean Stew

The beans and avocados in this recipe contain magnesium.

1 Tbsp. olive oil

1 cup onion, chopped into small pieces

2/3 cup couscous

2 cups vegetable broth

2 cups canned black beans, drained

1 tsp. canned chipotle in adobo, minced

28 oz. can stewed tomatoes

1 avocado, cubed into small pieces

1 or 2 green onions, sliced thin

4 Tbsp. low-fat, all-natural sour cream or yogurt

In a medium saucepan, sauté the onions and couscous in oil over medium heat for five minutes. Add broth, beans, chipotle, and tomatoes, cover and boil until couscous is tender, about five minutes. Serve with avocado, onions and sour cream on top. Serves four.

CHAPTER ELEVEN: Phosphorous

USDA/DRI: 700 mg/day

Phosphorous is the second most abundant element in the body after calcium. Ideally, the mineral makes up about half the amount of calcium in the bones, but in the standard American diet the consumption of high-phosphorous items like carbonated beverages and meat products may contribute to calcium deficiency. Phosphorous is important in bone and teeth formation, as well as most biochemical reactions in the body. Like calcium, it is also important in energy production and in enzyme function. It also has a role in kidney function and maintaining the acid-base balance in the body. Phosphorous is involved in muscle contraction, such as the heart muscle and helps nerve conduction.

According to Haas (1992), "a balance of calcium and phosphorous is also important in the prevention of arthritis, tooth and gum problems, stress, and cancer" (p.176).

The long-term use of antacids containing aluminum may deplete the body of phosphorous and calcium. Iron may also decrease the absorption of this mineral.

Food sources of phosphorous include meat and dairy products, seeds and nuts, 100% whole grains and most fruits and vegetables.

Whole Wheat Pasta with Chicken, Pesto and Sun-Dried Tomatoes

Pine nuts, chicken, and wheat contain phosphorous.

¾ lb. 100% whole wheat pasta

2 chicken breasts, grilled

¼ cup julienne sun-dried tomatoes

Pesto sauce:

½ bunch basil leaves

3 garlic cloves

½ cup pine nuts

¼ cup olive oil

¼ cup milk or half-and-half

½ cup parmesan cheese

Prepare pasta according to package directions. In a medium skillet or barbeque, grill the chicken over medium heat until cooked through (about five minutes on each side). Let the meat rest for five minutes, and then slice into strips. Meanwhile, make pesto sauce. Place all of the ingredients except oil and milk into a blender or food processor. After basil, garlic and nuts are blended, slowly stream olive oil into the processor, while the machine is running. Lastly, stream in the milk until sauce is smooth and creamy. Add to pasta, chicken and sun-dried tomatoes. Serves four.

CHAPTER TWELVE: Potassium

USDA/DRI: 4.7 grams/day

The sodium/potassium balance in the body is as important as the balance between calcium/phosphorous/magnesium. Too much sodium and a lack of potassium can lead to high blood pressure. Diuretic medication that is prescribed for high blood pressure can lead to decreased potassium and continued hypertension. The body naturally contains more potassium than sodium, but the standard American diet is full of processed food with an overabundance of sodium added to products. Vomiting and diarrhea also contribute to potassium loss, which is why healthcare practitioners sometimes recommend drinking beverages with electrolytes after these types of illnesses since they contain potassium. As with other nutrients, some potassium is lost in the cooking process.

Potassium supports nerve function and helps to regulate heart rhythm and blood pressure. It, along with sodium generates the electricity needed for nerve impulses, which is called the sodium-potassium pump, and is important in muscle contraction and the regulation of the heartbeat, as well as in the acid-base and water balances in the body. Potassium also contributes to protein synthesis and carbohydrate metabolism.

Food sources of potassium include apples, arugula, avocadoes, bananas, broccoli, chilies, citrus, lettuce, mushrooms, pears, potatoes (with skin), spinach, tomatoes, 100% whole grains, seeds, nuts, meat and fish.

Tomato Bruschetta on Toast

The tomatoes and wheat in this recipe contain potassium.

5 large tomatoes, chopped into small chunks

¼ cup basil leaves, minced

3 garlic cloves, minced

¼ red onion, minced

¼ cup olive oil

¼ cup balsamic vinegar

½ tsp. each: salt, pepper and oregano

1 100% whole grain baguette, sliced

Toss all ingredients together and let sit for an hour. Brush bread slices with olive oil or top with low-fat mozzarella, if desired and toast baguette slices in broiler or toaster oven for approximately three minutes, until golden brown. Top each slice with two or three tablespoons of bruschetta and serve. Makes eight servings.

Arugula Salad with Lemon Dressing

Arugula, chicken and lemons contain potassium.

1 bunch of arugula, washed

2 chicken breasts, grilled

¼ red onion, sliced into half-moon shapes

1 carrot, shredded

I can artichoke hearts in water, drained

¼ cup feta cheese

8 dolmas (grape leaves stuffed with rice-found in food specialty stores)

Lemon vinaigrette

Dressing:

¼ cup extra virgin olive oil

1 lemon, juiced

1 garlic clove, minced

½ tsp. salt and pepper

Sauté chicken over medium heat until thoroughly cooked (about five minutes on each side) and set aside. Put all of the dressing ingredients except oil into a wide-mouth jar. Slowly stream in the oil while whisking briskly to emulsify. Assemble the salad ingredients and add dressing. Serves four.

CHAPTER THIRTEEN: Sodium

USDA/DRI: 1.3-1.5 grams/day

Sodium is found in every cell in the body. Along with potassium and chloride, it is one of the electrolytes and helps to regulate the fluid balance of the body. It also regulates the fluid volume of the blood. It helps produce hydrochloric acid in the stomach for digestion, and is important in muscle contraction, nerve conduction, and the transportation of amino acids into the blood. Since it is one of the components of salt (40% sodium, 60% chloride), and salt is abundant in the standard American diet, it is rare to experience a sodium deficiency, but quite common to eat too much sodium, which may lead to high blood pressure and contribute to premenstrual problems. Some people are more sensitive to sodium than others, and there is some debate in the medical field regarding whether it is only salt intake, or if it is the balance of sodium and potassium that causes hypertension in some people. As mentioned in earlier chapters, research shows that too little potassium and magnesium in the body can also cause hypertension.

At any rate, cultures that eat much less processed foods and less salt have less problems relating to high blood pressure. Because it is important for body functioning, most recipes in the book incorporate salt for seasoning, but it can be left out of any meal if sodium intake is a concern.

Food sources of sodium include seafood and seaweed, beef, poultry, celery, beets, carrots, and artichokes.

Artichokes with Lemon Aioli

Artichokes and salt contain sodium.

4 large artichokes, cleaned and trimmed

¼ cup all-natural real mayonnaise

1 garlic clove, minced

Juice of half a lemon

Salt and pepper to taste

In a large stockpot, boil the artichokes in six cups of water until the leaves come off easily, approximately forty minutes. Meanwhile, combine the mayonnaise, garlic, lemon, salt and pepper. Drain the artichokes and serve with the aioli. Makes four servings as a side dish.

Beef Stew

Beef, celery and carrots are sources of sodium.

2.5 lbs. lean beef stew meat, cubed into 2" pieces

1 cup all-purpose flour

1/3 cup olive oil (plus more if needed)

2 large onions, chopped into small pieces

2 Tbsp. all-natural ketchup

1 cup dry red wine

2-3 potatoes cubed into 2" pieces

2 carrots, chopped into small chunks

4 cups all-natural beef broth

1 bay leaf

Salt and pepper to taste

Coat the beef in the flour. Place the oil and meat in a large stock pot over medium heat and brown a few pieces at a time, adding more oil if necessary. Remove browned meat from the pan. Add the onions to the pot and cook over medium heat until tender, about six minutes. Stir in ketchup and coat the onions. Pour the wine into the skillet and scrape up any browned bits; then add the beef to the onions. Stir in the potatoes, carrots, broth, bay leaf, salt and pepper. Cover and bring to a boil. Reduce heat and simmer for one-two hours until vegetables are tender. Serves six.

CHAPTER FOURTEEN: Sulfur

USDA/DRI: none

Sulfur is part of certain amino acids and B vitamins. It is important in protein synthesis and in enzyme reactions. It helps form collagen and is part of insulin, which is important for carbohydrate metabolism. The sulfur-containing amino acids also help form important antioxidants in the body. Ointments containing sulfur are also available for treating skin conditions such as eczema, psoriasis, and dermatitis.

Sulfur deficiency and toxicity are not a concern, except where the soil is depleted from this mineral. Modern day farming technology can deplete the soil from naturally occurring minerals, which in turn can reduce the amount of vitamins and minerals obtained from the food in which it is grown.

Food sources of sulfur include protein such as meats, fish, poultry, eggs, milk and legumes. Also, onions, garlic, cabbage, Brussels sprouts and turnips contain sulfur.

Tomato, Prosciutto and Lentil Soup

The ham, lentils, onions and garlic in this recipe contain sulfur.

1 cup lentils, washed and picked over

6 cups all-natural chicken broth

1-15 oz. can diced tomatoes

4 oz. prosciutto

½ onion, chopped into small pieces

4 cloves garlic, minced

½ tsp. cumin

⅛ tsp. oregano

2 Tbsp. olive oil

1 Tbsp. red wine vinegar

¼ tsp. hot sauce

Salt and pepper to taste

Combine all of the ingredients from the lentils to oregano, and bring to a boil uncovered, over medium high heat. Reduce heat to low and cook until lentils are tender, about one hour. Stir occasionally. In a small bowl whisk together the olive oil, vinegar, and hot sauce. Stir into the soup and warm for five minutes. Add salt and pepper, if desired. Serve with crusty 100% whole grain bread and a garden salad for a complete meal. Serves six.

CHAPTER FIFTEEN: Silicon

USDA/DRI: none

Silicon is the most abundant mineral in the earth's soil, since it is found in rock crystals. Likewise, it helps keep body systems strong, such as in connective tissue, nails, cartilage, bone, blood vessels, and tendons.

More research is needed since this element has only been studied for the last forty years or so. Haas (1992) believes that "a deficiency may cause decreased growth in bones and teeth, and increased risk for atherosclerosis and heart disease" (p.185).

Sources of silicon include wheat, oat and rice hulls, alfalfa, lettuce, cucumbers, avocados, strawberries, onions, and dark greens.

Spinach Crepes

Spinach, wheat, and onions contain silicon.

Filling:

1 Tbsp. butter

8 oz. white mushrooms, sliced

1 onion, chopped into small pieces

1 box frozen spinach, thawed and drained

2 garlic cloves, minced

2 Tbsp. lemon juice

1tsp. ground nutmeg

Salt and pepper to taste

12 oz. light all-natural cream cheese, cut into 6 pieces

Crepes:

2 eggs

2½ cups low-fat milk

2½ cups all purpose wheat flour

2 Tbsp. melted butter

To make the filling, melt the butter over medium heat, add the mushrooms and onions and sauté until softened, about six minutes. Place spinach in a clean kitchen towel and wring until the liquid is removed. Add the spinach, garlic, salt and pepper to the mushrooms and onions and heat through. Remove vegetable mixture from heat and place in a colander in the sink to drain the excess liquid. Return the vegetable mixture to the pan over medium heat and add the lemon, nutmeg and cream cheese. Stir until blended and remove from the heat.

Preheat the oven to warm. Beat the eggs and milk in a large bowl. Add the flour in small amounts and continue to beat. The batter will be thin, with a consistency like cream.

Brush a small frying pan with melted butter and place over medium-high heat. Pour ¼ cup of crepe batter into the bottom of the pan, and immediately rotate the pan so that the batter covers the bottom surface and the crepes are very thin. Turn the crepes once the edges start to separate from the pan and brown the other side. Place finished crepes in the oven to keep warm until all of the crepes are finished. Fill each crepe with about ¼ cup of vegetable filling and roll up. Serves eight.

CHAPTER SIXTEEN: Chromium

USDA/DRI: 20-35 mg/day

A very small amount of chromium (thus, it is considered an ultra-trace mineral) is necessary for carbohydrate metabolism and insulin function. As a result, it is thought to be important in diabetes prevention. Chromium has also been shown to lower LDL (bad) cholesterol and increase HDL (good) cholesterol levels in the blood. It is also linked to a reduction of atherosclerosis—perhaps due to its affect on cholesterol. According to Lieberman and Bruning (1997), it is noted that in Eastern cultures where low serum cholesterol levels are common, there are higher levels of chromium in the body. This is thought to be a result of higher levels of the mineral in the soil, and a diet that is less-processed and therefore, more chromium-rich. Much of the chromium in whole grains and sugarcane is lost in the refinement process, and it is not one of the nutrients usually added back in the enrichment phase. Also, a diet consisting of high amounts of refined flour and sugar products may even deplete the levels of chromium in the body, and it is known that the regular consumption of these products is linked to diabetes as well. Additionally, the chromium picolinate supplement has been shown to be effective in increasing muscle mass and reducing fat mass, but so far this is not conclusively proven.

Toxicity is not a problem since high levels are excreted by the body, but deficiency is a major concern. According to Lieberman and Bruning (1997), "approximately 80% of the population is deficient" (p. 199). This is probably due to the poor mineral content of the soil, as well as the detrimental standard American diet.

Sources of chromium include Brewer's yeast, beef, liver, 100% whole grains, oysters, potatoes, green peppers, chilies, eggs, chicken, apples, butter, bananas, and spinach.

Grandma Jo's Mashed Potatoes

The potatoes in this recipe, and the bananas in the

following recipe contain chromium.

5 lb. bag of russet potatoes, peeled and chopped into large chunks

½ cup milk, plus more if needed

1 stick butter

Salt and pepper to taste

Boil the potatoes until tender, approximately thirty minutes.

Add milk and butter and mash together to desired

creaminess/lumpiness. Serves ten people as a side dish.

Flax Banana Bread

1½ cups all-purpose flour

½ cup ground flaxseed

¾ cup sugar

1 tsp. baking powder

½ tsp. baking soda

½ tsp. salt

2 eggs

1/3 cup vegetable oil

1 cup mashed ripe bananas

Topping:

¼ cup packed brown sugar

½ tsp. ground cinnamon

Preheat oven to 350°F. Spray 8 ½ x 4 ½-inch loaf pan with cooking spray. Mix together flour, flaxseed, sugar, baking powder, baking soda and salt. In another bowl, beat together the eggs and oil. Add the flour mixture and bananas to the egg mixture, stirring until dry ingredients are moistened (mixture will be sticky). Spoon batter into the prepared pan, spreading evenly. Mix topping ingredients and sprinkle over the batter. Pat gently into batter. Bake until toothpick inserted in center comes out clean, about one hour. Cool in pan for fifteen minutes, and then turn bread onto wire rack to cool completely. Serve with jelly, honey, butter or plain. Makes

eight slices.

CHAPTER SEVENTEEN: Cobalt

USDA/DRI: none

Cobalt is an important part of vitamin B-12. Cobalt is essential in red blood cell production and in forming nerve function. Radioactive cobalt-60 is used to treat certain cancers. According to Haas (1992), "too much cobalt can adversely affect people, possibly causing thyroid and heart problems, and increased activity in the bone marrow" (p. 190). This is an example of how too much of even a healthy nutrient can be detrimental to health.

Food sources of cobalt include meat, liver, kidneys, clams, oysters, fish, milk, legumes, spinach, cabbage, lettuce, beet greens, and figs.

Grandma Jo's Cole Slaw

The cabbage in this recipe, and the meat and beans in the following recipe contain cobalt.

1 head cabbage, shredded

1 cup all-natural real mayonnaise

¼ cup apple cider vinegar

1-2 tsp. sugar

Salt and pepper to taste

In large bowl, add the salt and pepper to the shredded cabbage. In a separate bowl, whisk together mayonnaise, vinegar and sugar to a thin consistency, adding more if needed. It should taste slightly tangy and sweet. Add the dressing to the cabbage and toss. Cover and refrigerate for an hour or more. Serves six as a side dish.

Reda's Chili

2 lbs. lean ground beef

1 large onion, chopped

1 quart of tomato sauce

2 cans pinto beans

2 cans kidney beans

1 bottle of beer

2 Tbsp. chili powder

2 garlic cloves, minced

½ tsp. each: salt, pepper, oregano and cumin

In a large stock pot, brown onions and ground beef together over medium heat until meat is nearly cooked through, approximately ten minutes. Add tomatoes, beer and seasonings to meat mixture and simmer for two hours or until the taste of alcohol has been eliminated. Add the beans and simmer for an additional thirty minutes. Serve with cornbread, chopped onions and/or grated cheddar cheese. Serves eight.

CHAPTER EIGHTEEN: Copper

USDA/DRI: 900 mcg/day

Copper is essential to make hemoglobin, in energy production and in cell respiration. It also supports vitamin C and works with it to form collagen, tissues and bones. In addition, copper is important in fighting free radicals, is involved in producing melanin, and is believed to help treat arthritis as an anti-inflammatory agent. Like most metals, it is a conductor of electricity, so it helps nervous system function.

A copper deficiency is thought to be rare, but with the prevalence of processed foods stripped of their vitamins and minerals, it is possible that many Americans are experiencing a lack of this beneficial mineral. However, overdosing could be just as dangerous: according to Lieberman and Bruning (1997), "excessive doses of copper produce nausea, vomiting, abdominal pains, diarrhea, headache, dizziness, and a metallic taste in the mouth. If untreated, this can lead to death" (p. 163). Again, it is important to eat a balanced diet with a wide variety of healthy foods—and not to over consume anything, even if it is a healthy item.

Sources of copper include 100% whole grains, shellfish, liver, peas, beans, nuts, oysters, soybeans, leafy greens, dried fruits, cocoa, black pepper and yeast. Also, the use of copper pipes and cookware increase intake of this mineral.

Peanut and Rice Soup

This may not sound as delicious as it is. If you love tomatoes and peanuts, you will love the smooth taste, and the rice makes it a hearty meal. The peanuts in this recipe provide copper.

2 tsp. peanut oil

1 garlic clove, minced

1 28-oz. can chopped tomatoes

½ cup creamy all-natural peanut butter

8 cups all-natural chicken broth

1 Tbsp. balsamic vinegar

¼ tsp. cayenne

1 cup cooked brown rice

6 scallions, sliced thin

¼ cup salted peanuts, chopped

Salt and pepper to taste

In a large stockpot, sauté the oil and garlic over medium heat for one minute. Add the tomatoes, peanut butter, broth, vinegar, cayenne, salt and pepper, and whisk to combine. Bring to a boil. Reduce to low, cover and simmer for twenty minutes. Add the rice and heat through. Ladle into bowls and garnish with scallions and peanuts. Serves six.

CHAPTER NINETEEN: Iodine

USDA/DRI: 150 mcg/day

Iodine is vital for healthy thyroid hormone function and for maintaining the body's basal metabolic rate, which is the measure of the body's use of energy. The thyroid affects reproductive health, mental and physical growth, nerve, muscle and bone formation, circulation, and the metabolism of all nutrients. A lack of thyroid hormone (hypothyroidism) may cause problems in these areas, as well as weight gain and fatigue. Haas (1992) suggests that "iodine deficiency increases the risk of breast, ovary, and uterine cancer and may be a part of the cause of fibrocystic breast disease" (p. 196). The classic condition of iodine deficiency is called goiter, in which the thyroid gland becomes enlarged in order to compensate for insufficient hormone production. In fact, in locations where soil levels of iodine are low, goiter is more common and these areas are referred to as "goiter belts." In the

United States, these areas include the Midwest, Pacific Northwest and Great Lakes regions.

Sources of iodine include ocean fish, kelp, iodized salt, onions, mushrooms, lettuce, spinach, green peppers, pineapple, peanuts, cheddar cheese, and 100% whole wheat products. Sushi would be a great source of iodine too.

Portobello Mushroom Spinach Pitas

The spinach, mushrooms and wheat in this recipe contain iodine.

2 Portobello mushrooms

¼ red onion, sliced into half-moon shapes

1 bunch fresh spinach

2-100% whole wheat pitas, foccacia or flat bread

½ cup light shredded mozzarella

2 garlic cloves, minced

2 tsp. Italian seasoning

2 tsp. olive oil

¼ cup balsamic vinegar

Cooking spray

Salt and pepper to taste

Preheat the oven broiler. Wash (many chefs say not to wash mushrooms, but unless you buy only organic mushrooms, I think it's still a good idea to give them a rinse) and slice mushrooms and onions and place them in a shallow baking pan. Spray the vegetables with vegetable oil and sprinkle with Italian seasoning. Pour balsamic vinegar over the vegetables and toss. Broil for approximately eight minutes. Check and stir as needed.

Meanwhile heat the olive oil over medium heat. Sauté the garlic and spinach until spinach is wilted, approximately five minutes.

Remove the vegetables from oven. Spray the pitas with vegetable oil and top with ¼ cup mozzarella cheese. Broil for two minutes until the cheese is melted. Top the pitas with mushrooms, onions, spinach and serve. Serves two.

CHAPTER TWENTY: Iron

USDA/DRI: 8-18 mg/day

Iron forms hemoglobin in the blood, which is the oxygen-carrying component of red blood cells. Red blood cells take oxygen from the lungs and distribute it into the other tissues of the body. Similarly, iron forms myoglobin, which holds oxygen and carries it into the muscles. Iron is also needed for energy production and protein metabolism.

Anemia, fatigue, lack of stamina, headaches, dizziness, difficulty swallowing, heart palpitations during exertion, weakened immunity, paleness, apathy, irritability, and poor memory are all indicators of iron deficiency. According to Lieberman and Bruning (1997), "iron deficiency is the most common nutritional deficiency in the world with vast numbers of people becoming deficient at some point in their lives" (p.156).

Iron can be difficult to absorb in the body, and it works best with adequate levels of other nutrients like vitamins A, B and antioxidants. Items like coffee, tea and antacids may interfere with iron absorption. On the other hand, tomato products assist the body with iron absorption.

Sources of iron include 100% whole grains, beef, liver, pork, lamb, chicken, shellfish, egg yolks, brown rice, legumes, mushrooms, nuts, seeds, green leafy vegetables, and dried fruits.

Fried Brown Rice

This is a recipe I use a lot when I have leftover meat and rice. The meat, egg, and brown rice in this recipe contain iron.

6 oz. leftover meat, such as chicken, pork or beef, chopped into small pieces

2 cups cooked brown rice (day-old is best)

2 eggs

½ cup frozen peas and carrots

1 garlic clove, minced

¼ onion, chopped into small pieces

1 Tbsp. sesame oil

½ cup soy sauce

Salt and pepper to taste

In a wok or large skillet, sauté the onion in the sesame oil over medium heat until tender, about five minutes. Add the garlic and sauté for one-two minutes. Add the frozen vegetables and heat through. Meanwhile, make space in the wok to scramble the eggs, then mix with all of the vegetables. Add the rice, meat and soy sauce and heat through. A full meal could be made with the addition of a side of spring rolls or pot stickers, and a salad topped with the carrot-miso dressing in Chapter One. Serves four.

CHAPTER TWENTY-ONE: Manganese

USDA/DRI: 1.8-2.3 mg/day

Manganese helps the body use vitamins, protein, cholesterol and fatty acids. It is also useful in glucose metabolism, nerve function, reproduction, bone health and in energy production. It is used in the body as an antioxidant—fighting free radicals as part of the superoxide dismutase (SOD) enzyme. There is not much risk for manganese toxicity, although in areas like Chile where it is mined, workers have been at risk to develop a syndrome called *locura manganica* (manganese madness), which, Haas (1992) states "is characterized by mania leading to anorexia, weakness and apathy" (p. 208). At the other extreme, Eades (1994) wrote that "manganese deficiency can lead to fragile bones, rashes, sugar intolerance, high cholesterol, nausea, weight loss, and reproductive problems" (p. 100). Unless a person is exposed to high amounts of manganese via inhalation, the health benefits of manganese outweigh the risks of toxicity.

Food sources of manganese include nuts, 100% whole grains, egg yolks, seeds, spinach, legumes, leafy greens, alfalfa, black tea and coffee.

Spinach Lasagna

The spinach and whole grains in this recipe both contain manganese. To incorporate additional manganese, add a handful of toasted pine nuts to the recipe.

12 oz. 100% whole wheat lasagna noodles

1 bunch fresh spinach, washed and trimmed

1 lb. cremini or white mushrooms sliced

1 Tbsp. olive oil

2 cups low-fat ricotta cheese

2 cups low-fat mozzarella cheese

3 cups Italian tomato sauce (recipe follows)

Preheat oven to 350°F. While the sauce is cooking, sauté the mushrooms in olive oil over medium heat until tender, about six minutes. Add spinach and sauté until wilted, about five minutes.

Put a ladleful of sauce into the bottom of a 13x9 pan. Layer uncooked noodles over the sauce (the noodles will cook in the oven). Spoon more sauce over the noodles and scoop half of the ricotta and mozzarella on top. Scoop half of the vegetable mixture on top of the cheese. Make another layer of noodles, sauce, cheese and vegetables. Top with noodles, sauce and the rest of the mozzarella. Place foil tightly over pan and bake for about 45 minutes. Remove the foil and bake an additional fifteen minutes. Remove from oven and let cool ten-fifteen minutes before serving. Serves ten.

Italian Tomato Sauce

1 large onion, chopped into small pieces

3 garlic cloves, minced

1 Tbsp. olive oil

1 quart canned stewed tomatoes

1 quart canned tomato sauce

1 Tbsp. tomato paste

1 Tbsp. honey

1 tsp. each: salt, pepper, and Italian seasoning

Sauté the garlic and onion in oil over medium heat until tender, about six minutes. Add the tomatoes, sauce, paste and seasonings, and gently simmer for at least thirty minutes. Add the honey and simmer an additional twenty minutes. Taste and add additional seasonings as desired.

CHAPTER TWENTY-TWO: Molybdenum

USDA/DRI: 45 mcg/day

Molybdenum is important in enzyme production, uric acid formation and iron utilization. Haas (1992) also believes that it is "an important nutrient in carbohydrate metabolism and sulfite and nitrosamine detoxification" (p. 210). Sulfites and nitrosamines are preservatives that are used in some meats, cheese, beer and wine and have been linked to certain cancers. Uric acid is a byproduct of protein metabolism that is important for good health, but too much uric acid can cause gout, which links too much molybdenum in the body to this painful problem.

Some of the toxicity problems associated with this mineral may be caused by a deficiency in copper because the two minerals compete in the body for absorption. Molybdenum deficiency is common, due the depletion of nutrients in agricultural soil, and may cause vision problems, rapid breathing and a rapid heartbeat.

Sources of molybdenum include 100% whole grains (especially the germ), oats, buckwheat and wheat germ, legumes, potatoes, spinach, cauliflower, peas and soybeans.

Oatmeal Fruit Crisp

The oats in this recipe contain molybdenum.

Filling:

3 cups sliced peeled fresh pears or apples

¼ cup sugar

1 Tbsp. all-purpose flour

Topping:

1/3 cup uncooked, quick-cooking oats

3 Tbsp. packed brown sugar

2 Tbsp. all-purpose flour

½ tsp. ground cinnamon

¼ tsp. salt

2 Tbsp. cold butter, cut into pieces

Preheat oven to 375°F. Spray an eight-inch square baking pan with cooking spray. In a medium bowl, combine filling ingredients and spoon into the pan. In a small bowl, combine oats, brown sugar, flour, cinnamon and salt. Cut in the butter until mixture resembles coarse crumbs. Sprinkle topping evenly over filling. Bake until the edges are bubbly, approximately thirty minutes. Serve warm with low-fat vanilla ice cream, if desired. Serves six.

CHAPTER TWENTY-THREE: Selenium

USDA/DRI: 55 mcg/day

Selenium helps activate the antioxidant enzyme,

glutathione peroxidase, so it contributes to protection from aging

diseases such as cancer and cardiovascular disease. It is one of the

many nutrients whose soil levels have been depleted from modern

farming practices, and it is widely recognized that low soil levels

of selenium are related to higher cancer rates. Haas (1992)

declares that "South Dakota has the highest soil levels of selenium

in the United States, and Ohio has the lowest. Notably, Ohio has

more than twice the amount of cancer than South Dakota" (p. 212).

Due to its important role as an antioxidant, deficiency may cause

an increased risk for cancer, cardiovascular disease, hypertension,

and strokes.

Keshan disease (a heart condition in China where the soil

levels of selenium are low) is possibly caused by selenium

deficiency, since supplementation of this mineral has helped sufferers of this condition. Selenium also seems to protect form heavy metals and may aid in protein synthesis, growth, and fertility (especially in the males).

Sources of selenium include Brewer's yeast, wheat germ, liver, butter, fish, Brazil nuts, shellfish, garlic onions, mushrooms, broccoli, tomatoes, radishes, and Swiss chard.

Portobello Wrap

The wheat, garlic, onions and mushrooms in these wraps contain selenium.

2 Portobello mushrooms, washed and sliced

¼ red onion, sliced into half-moon shapes

2 garlic cloves, minced

¼ cup julienne sun-dried tomatoes

2 large leafs of romaine or other lettuce

2-100% whole grain (or any kind) of high fiber wraps

½ cup low-fat shredded mozzarella

2 Tbsp. olive oil

2 Tbsp. balsamic vinegar

1 Tbsp. pesto sauce (recipe, Chapter Eleven)

Salt and pepper to taste

Preheat oven broiler. Wash and slice the mushrooms, garlic and onions and place into a shallow baking pan. Toss vegetables with the oil, vinegar and seasonings. Broil in the oven for approximately eight minutes. Check and stir as needed. Heat the wraps directly over open flame or in the microwave for ten seconds each. Spread pesto sauce on the wrap, layer lettuce, tomatoes and cheese. Scoop mushroom mixture into wrap, roll up and serve. Serves two.

CHAPTER TWENTY-FOUR: Zinc

USDA/DRI: 8-11 mg/day

Zinc is a necessary element in over one hundred enzymes. It is important in immune system function, which is why many natural cold remedies are made of it, and it seems to speed healing for surgery and burn patients. It helps normal development and sexual function, especially related to the prostate and semen. Low zinc levels may cause pregnancy complications, miscarriage and birth defects. A deficiency may also lead to sexual dysfunction, which as Lieberman and Bruning (1997) point out, is perhaps why oysters are considered an aphrodisiac—they are high in zinc (p151). Zinc also detoxifies certain chemicals in the body, and helps metabolize carbohydrates. It is important in energy production and the synthesis of DNA, as well as in the treatment of skin problems. As with selenium and chromium, much of it comes from the soil, so it is important to keep farm land healthy and rich with these natural minerals. Since zinc comes from whole grains, processing the flour will eliminate the zinc, as it is not added back during the enrichment process.

Zinc deficiency may cause slowed growth and sexual development, lowered immunity, fatigue, poor appetite, learning disabilities, acne, skin problems, white spots on the nails, and possibly sterility. One of the early signs of zinc deficiency is a loss of taste, which is dangerous for elderly people especially, since this may contribute to a lack of appetite and proper nutrition.

Food sources of zinc include animal foods, especially oysters, 100% whole grains, beans, nuts ginger, mustard, pepper, peas, carrots, beets, and cabbage.

Whole Wheat Pasta with Pesto, Chicken, and Peas

The chicken, wheat and peas in this recipe contain zinc.

1 lb.-100% whole wheat pasta

2 chicken breasts, grilled

1 Tbsp. olive oil

½ cup frozen peas, thawed to room temperature

Pesto sauce (recipe, Chapter Eleven)

Prepare pasta according to package directions. In a medium skillet, sauté the chicken in olive oil over medium heat until cooked through (about five minutes on each side). Let rest, and then slice into strips. Add to pasta, and toss with pesto and peas. Serves four.

CONCLUSION

After reading this cookbook, it is easy to see why these essential nutrients are so important since they all perform vital functions for good health. Now imagine what a diet devoid of these nutritious vitamins and minerals does to the body. Without calcium, the heart would not beat properly and the skeletal system would disintegrate. Without vitamin C, people would eventually develop scurvy and possibly die. Without a balanced diet with a wide variety of good healthy food, people would be missing out on all of the benefits mentioned in this book, in addition to untold benefits yet to be discovered. It is easy to understand why many people who consume only packaged, processed and fast foods have problems with obesity and poor health quality.

Some additional powerful benefits in whole foods include antioxidants (as mentioned in several chapters), which fight age-related diseases such as the three killers mentioned in the introduction: cardiovascular disease, diabetes, and cancer, plus many more health problems. Antioxidants may protect body cells from damage caused by the oxidative effects of free radicals. Free radicals are formed by many things, including smoking, pollution, and by consuming too much processed food.

Fresh food also contains phytochemicals (beneficial plant compounds such as carotenoids and flavonoids), trace elements and other benefits. In fact, there are so many benefits to eating wholesome natural food that the nutritional community continues to discover beneficial properties, which is why one of America's top oncologists, Dr. Larry Norton has stated, "God put a lot more good stuff in an apple than I know about" (ABC: The View, Oct. 2005).

Not only do fresh fruits and vegetables provide all of the health benefits discussed previously, but also fiber which is vital to healthy living. Fiber helps to maintain a healthy digestive tract, and it helps to prevent high blood pressure, heart disease, stroke, some cancers and diabetes. Plus, it is beneficial to add as many flavors and textures to a menu so that readers do not have to rely on fat or sugar for flavor.

As mentioned previously, whole grains are also essential to a healthy diet, and are a good source of fiber and other nutrients. It is important, however, to look for grains that are listed as 100% whole grain or 100% whole wheat. According to Roizen and Oz (2006):

> Whole grain means that the grain still has all three of its original elements: the outer shell or bran, which contains fiber and B vitamins; the germ, which contains phytochemicals and B vitamins; and the endosperm, which contains carbohydrates and protein. (p.256)

Unfortunately, many packaged and fast foods contain white or enriched flour, and even what is called "wheat flour," but if it is not listed as 100%, it is devoid of grain's health benefits, and may in fact, be harmful to health if consumed in excess.

The good new for busy families is that there are some healthy "convenience" foods in the market. For example, a great staple of any pantry is canned tomato sauce (most are minimally processed), which is full of lycopene, a nutrient that fights cancer, especially of the prostate. Frozen and canned produce are usually a decent choice when fresh is not available, since most vegetables and fruit are frozen and canned immediately after harvesting and sometimes, blanching, which does not deplete all of its nutrients. There are also high-fiber cereals, oatmeal and bread (again, 100% whole grain), as well as nuts, vegetable and meat stocks, bottled water and whole fruit juice, among others. The healthiest items are found in their whole form, without a lot of additives and preservatives, sugar and salt. So by reading the labels, most ingredients will be recognizable, without a lot of foreign chemical ingredients. After awhile of eating fresh wholesome food, it is harder to subsist solely on the standard American diet of fast or packaged food. The standard American diet lacks a variety of taste and texture that a varied diet provides. It is important to eat a variety of nutritious food due to the fact that many of the nutrients in this cookbook function best when there are adequate levels of other nutrients in the body. Also, remember that it is more important to eat natural whole foods, even if they are canned or frozen than it is to avoid them altogether if you don't have the time to prepare fresh food.

Another important fact to mention is that it is more important than ever to nourish the body due to the current state of the environment. Like mentioned in previous chapters, modern farming practices have a major impact on health, by depleting the soil of the nutrients needed to thrive. Organic produce is grown without chemical fertilizers and insecticides. Not only does it usually taste superior to conventionally grown items, it tends to contain higher levels of nutrients since the soil is richer in nutrients from the natural compost used to fertilize it. Also pesticides can counteract the health benefits of fresh food. Therefore, it is recommended that readers use organic produce, meat and dairy whenever possible. At any rate, according to Environmental Working Group (Environmental Working Group [EWG], 2007, The Full List: 43 Fruits & Veggies), there are food items that tend to contain more chemical pesticides than others, so it is important to eat these in their organic form, if possible. These include apples, celery, cherries, grapes, lettuce, nectarines, peaches, pears, potatoes, spinach, strawberries and bell peppers.

The human body is a miraculous, intricate system that requires a balance of diet and exercise to function at its peak. Without the proper balance of vitamins and minerals in the body disease, lack of energy, and a poorer quality of life would likely result. Hopefully this cookbook will be one in personal libraries that helps readers integrate whole foods into the diet and helps contribute to long, happy, and healthy lives.

REFERENCES

American Cancer Society (2006). Statistics for 2006. Retrieved
    August 10, 2006, from
    http://www.cancer.org/downloads/STT/CAFF2006PWSecu
    red.pdf

American Heart Association (2006). Heart disease and stroke
    statistics—2006 update. Retrieved July 6, 2006 from
    http://circ.ahajournals.org/cgi/content/short/113/6/e85

Eades, M.D. (1994). *The doctor's complete guide to vitamins and
    minerals.* New York: Dell Publishing.

Environmental Working Group (2007). The Full List: 43 Fruits &
    Veggies. Retrieved September 7, 2007 from
    http://www.foodnews.org/

Gower, T. (2006). Is diabetes in your future? *Natural Health,*
    July/August 2006, 51-52.

Haas, E. (1992). *Staying healthy with nutrition.* Berkeley: Celestial
    Arts.

Bruning, N., & Lieberman, S. (1997). *The real vitamin & mineral
    book.* Garden City Park: Avery Publishing Group.

National Diabetes Information Clearinghouse (2005). National
    diabetes statistics. Retrieved July 6, 2006 from
    http://diabetes.niddk.nih.gov/dm/pubs/statistics/index.htm#
    7

Norton, L. (2006). *The View.* Prod. ABC Daytime, Barwall
    Productions. ABC, New York.

NutritionData (2006). Nutrition facts & calorie counter. Retrieved
    July 27, 2006 from
    http://www.nutritiondata.com/index/html

Nutrition Information Resource Center (2001). Most frequently
    asked questions about RDAs and DRIs. Retrieved June 26,
    2006 from http://nal.usda.gov/fnic

Richter, H. (2002). *Fresh produce guide*. Apopka: Try Foods intl.

Roizen, M., & Oz, M. (2006). *You on a diet.* New York: Free
    Press.

Siple, M. (2005). Nourish: one delicious dinner features 10 top
    healing foods. *Natural Health*, March 2005, 61-67.

U.S. Department of Agriculture National Agricultural Library
    (2004). Dietary reference intakes: recommended intakes for
    individuals. Retrieved August 10, 2006 from
    http://www.iom.edu/Object.File/Master/21/372/0.pdf